What Others Are Saying About Youth Health Endurance: What Scientists Know and You Should Too!

WOW - What an eye-opening book!

William K. Penny (UK)
What an addictive read... I could not stop reading it. I'm sad that I reached the end, but there is just so much useful info in here, I know it will stay by the kitchen bench for a while.
I had no idea about half the potential dangers spoken of in this well-researched book. I have to say, if it weren't for the really helpful images, I may have gotten a little bogged down in some of the technical jargon.
Some really positive advice at the tail end of the book shows us how far we have come as humans... It's books like this one that help educate us all towards a better future!

Great Information and Entertaining

M. Schramski (USA)

I found YOUTH HEALTH ENDURANCE to be a great reminder of what we need to do to get and stay healthy. Written in a straight-forward way, anyone can understand the steps that the authors lay out to become a healthier person. I especially loved the retro ads that show how far food science has come. They gave me my chuckles for the day.

Science Meets Simplicity

Glenn Garnes (USA)

What I liked most about Youth Health Endurance was the simplicity it brings to a very important topic. I can't believe all the myths we've lived with over the years, promoted primarily by our government. It makes it even more important to stay plugged in to updated information. Youth Health Endurance makes it easy to do that. Loved the mind teaser towards the end of the book too.

Great Book!!!!

Katie (Hawaii)

This book was so great, it was written so I can actually understand what the Author was talking about rather than the usual science mumbo jumbo. I loved all the pictures and I loved how they were able to show how far we have come in science and medicine since the 20's. I highly recommend this book to anyone who is looking to improve their health and wellness.

A Fascinating New Book About Health & Aging!

bevsweb (Oregon)

The authors present compelling evidence of how to enjoy better health and live longer! It is presented in an easy to read and understandable format for the lay person.
This book provides a comprehensive look at our bodies from the cellular structure where disease begins and ends. As a layperson with no science background, I could easily grasp some difficult concepts and reason along with the authors how I can live longer and be free from most disease. A must read book I highly suggest for anyone concerned about their health and the aging process.

Makes me want to know more

Jennifer McGahan (Spicewood, TX United States)

Very intriguing information I've never heard before. I actually spent a lot of time looking over the resources the author provided. Exciting!

Great information to start you on your journey of a healthier life

Sigrid Gangsoy (Sydney, NSW, AU)

Being very interested in living a healthy life-style I thought the information in "Youth Health Endurance: What Scientists Know and You Should Too" gave a very informed and well written account of the structure of the basic cell and how it operates. It makes sense that if the very basic building blocks of our body are not performing at their very highest level then how can we expect to live life at our peak? Much like "spark plugs" - if they're not all operating at peak performance the car's performance is less than it should be. I'd recommend this book to anyone wanting more information on how our very basic cells work and the impact they have on our health if they are not.

Youth Health Endurance:

What Scientists Know and You Should Too!

Lorinda Snyder and David Prejean

I0116350

© 2012 Prejean Publishing

Palm Springs CA

Prejeanpublishing.com

ALL RIGHTS RESERVED. This book contains material protected under International and Federal Copyright Laws and Treaties. Any unauthorized reprint or use of this material is prohibited. No part of this book may be reproduced or transmitted in any form or by any means, electronic or mechanical, including photocopying, recording, or by any information storage and retrieval system without express written permission from the author / publisher.

Disclaimer and disclosure: Every effort has been made to provide accurate (as of this writing) information. All sources have been cited at the back of the book and you are encouraged to read and evaluate the information for yourself. None of the information as presented here has been evaluated by the FDA or any other agency. Nothing in this book should be construed as medical advice or replace medical advice. This information is not intended to diagnose, treat, cure or prevent any disease or other condition. All the sources of supply and information in this book are provided as a courtesy to the reader, the authors have no affiliation with any links or sources provided.

"The part can never be well unless the whole is well..."

~**Plato**

Introduction

Man's quest for good health goes back thousands of years. Health has been called the greatest of all wealth and most of us would agree. Poor health makes it very difficult to spend quality time with family and friends or to enjoy whatever level of financial abundance we have achieved.

Health care is an enormous industry, in the US alone, over three *trillion* dollars are spent each year trying to diagnose and treat poor health. That number will double by the year 2020. Stated another way, health care is one of the largest economies in the world.

Yet, with all that money being spent, we still rank 37th in the world as far as the health of our citizens, this puts the US in the same category as many third world nations. Chile, for example, spends an average of $270 per person annually (2009) for health care while we spend about $4000, yet Chileans are healthier.

To put this number into perspective, according to the documentary, *Thrive*, we could end world hunger for the bargain price of $280 billion dollars, just a portion of the money the US spends every year on health care now.

In 2005 the Centers for Disease Control issued a statement predicting that the generation born after 2000 will be the first generation in history to live shorter lives than their parents.

It estimated in that generation, one out of every three people will suffer from diabetes in adulthood; for minorities, the number is one out of two. It further predicted staggering rates of cardiovascular disease. The projected cost of health care for this generation is being called "insurmountable".

Why is that we spend more, but achieve less? Why are we sicker today with all the "miracle drugs" available to us?

When it comes to health, Plato could have more accurately have said, "the whole can never be well unless the parts are well." Since we are made up of cells, we are literally only as well as our sickest cell.

Information about things that increase health has always been a booming business, even if the information is incomplete, inaccurate, or even dangerously wrong. When it came to the attention of the US government about 70 years ago, that a percentage of the population was feeling "sluggish", it was determined that people were lacking thiamine in their diet. Always eager to help, the government published and distributed this advice:

Here are a few more examples of "health advice" that has been dispensed:

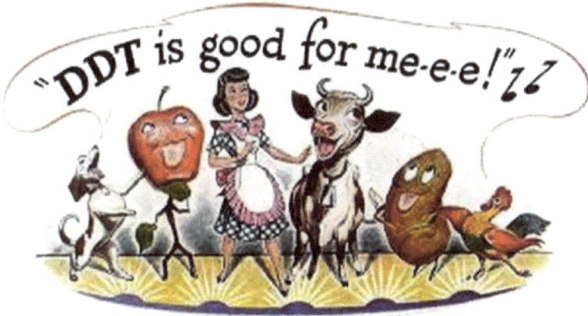

Seriously?

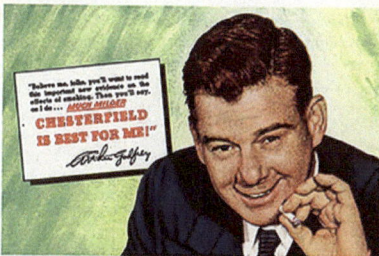

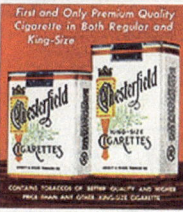

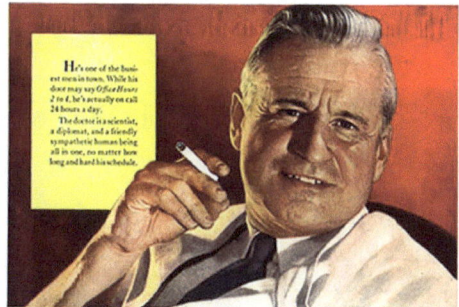

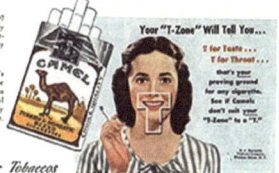

What mom wouldn't appreciate this wonderful suggestion:

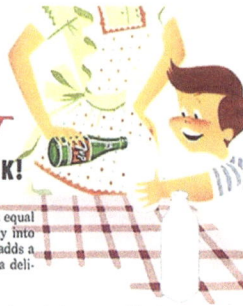

And to further promote the health and safety of America's children we have:

They're funny and shocking now. We wonder how anyone could have ever believed that donuts, cigarettes, DDT and lead paint were beneficial, but that was the accepted norm at the time and it would be several decades before the truth would be discovered.

It goes back to the search we talked about earlier. We know that ultimately the state of our health is largely in our own hands and we are eager to understand what makes us healthy and to do (at least some of) the things we need to do to preserve or restore our health. Unfortunately, that often leaves us vulnerable to misinformation or outright scams.

Fortunately, we have the benefit today of a few watchdog agencies who try to cut through a lot of the hype and provide factual information for us to use.

We also have the benefit of access to research findings through university libraries and the internet so we can educate ourselves and make informed decisions about our health and the health of our families.

Before now, we were in the same situation as the people who lived in the Dark Age in Europe who were not allowed to learn to read. All they were allowed to know about the world or God or anything else was what those in control wanted them to know. Anyone who dared to "peek behind the curtain" paid a very high price, often with their life.

Once people could find the information for themselves and make their own decisions about what to believe, Europe entered the Renaissance and beyond. This opened the doorway to questioning and searching for answers. That searching spawned one advancement after another, with intellectual pioneers building upon the work of one another to create the world of science the way we know it today.

We are on the brink of another Age of Enlightenment when it comes to health. We've come a long way from the time when disease was thought to have been caused by sin. There are astounding breakthroughs that have been made in the past ten years that have yet to make the national news, but are quietly changing the lives of the people who know about and implement them. One in particular is what we would call a Game Changer, something that will radically alter what we consider to be "normal aging" now and far into the future.

One of the things science has discovered is the adult brain learns best when new information is linked logically to information it has already processed and accepted. That is also the format of this book. We will start with a short refresher on cells and how they function. As you read over it, you'll find that most of it sounds very familiar, that's the part that's already been processed and accepted. The chapters after that will introduce the new information that will build upon what you already know and give you a clear understanding of what comprises this thing we call "health", that it's much more than the absence of disease, and how to implement this new knowledge.

A Quick Refresher on Cells

If you're anything like us, it's been awhile since you sat in high school biology class and learned about the structure and function of cells. Actually, there is so much new information that is just being discovered about cells and what they do, that even if you took a science class just last year, much of the information to come will still be new to you.

Each of us is the result of the collective effort of the sixty to ninety *trillion* cells that make up our body and its internal structures. There are enough cells in one human body that, placed end to end, they would circle the Earth four to five times. We look at ourselves and the people around us and see a single organism, but the truth is, we are a walking, talking, thinking, eating, breathing collection of cells.

We live and die at a cellular level. Just like an immense forest is only as healthy as the individual trees within it, we are only as healthy as each of our cells. All disease and degeneration can be traced to cellular damage. Again, we live and die at a cellular level. This simple fact is so important, you'll hear us say it several more times throughout this book.

Inside of a Cell

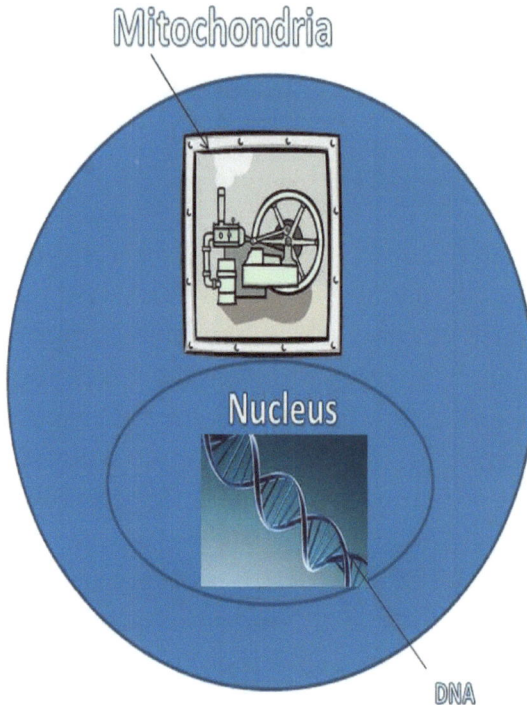

One of the structures found inside each cell is the mitochondria. Cells can have anywhere from 200 to 10,000 mitochondria each. The mitochondria is the power plant for the cell. It produces energy in the form of *adenosine triphosphate* or ATP. ATP contains three phosphate atoms and fuels the cells to perform every movement, process and function in the body. Without ATP, nothing would function and the entire body would quickly die.

During the process of producing ATP, the mitochondria also produces two types of very special molecules; *Reactive Oxygen Species* also known as ROS and *Reduced Species* or RS. Together, these molecules are known as *Redox Signaling Molecules*. Don't be surprised if you've never heard of either of these because when most of us were learning about biology, the thinking was that redox signaling molecules were simply by-products of ATP production and were eliminated as waste. Turns out, nothing could be further from the truth, but we'll get to that in a minute.

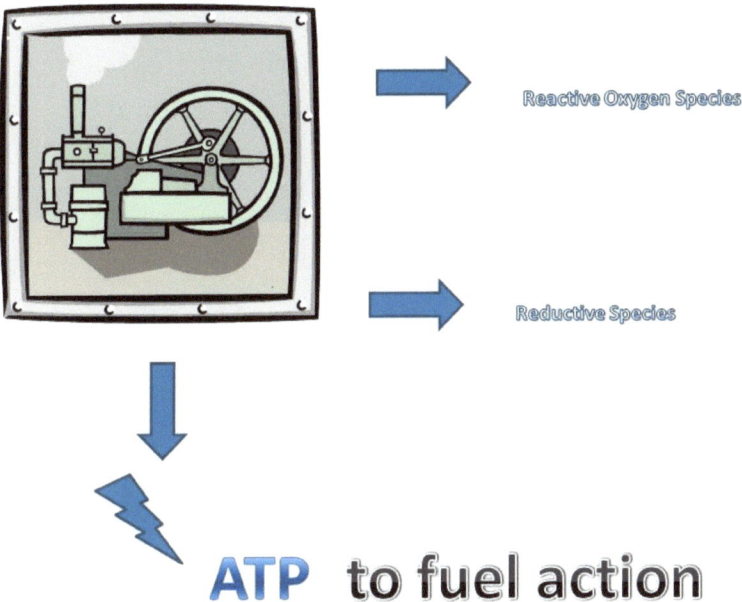

Reactive Oxygen Species

Reductive Species

ATP to fuel action

In the process of using ATP for energy, one of the phosphate atoms is "burned off" to provide the "spark" the cell needs to access the energy. It's very similar to the way your car uses spark plugs to combust the fuel and power the engine. The

ATP molecule then becomes ADP (*adenosine DI-phosphate* as opposed to it's original form, *adenosine TRI-phosphate*). The mighty mitochondria then "recycles" the molecule by attaching a new phosphate atom to it and sending it back out as ATP to be used again. This process is repeated millions of times every minute of every day. When we're doing something that requires endurance, we can give our mitochondria a helping hand by using a supplement like creatine which provides the extra phosphates the mitochondria needs in order to recycle the ATP faster and give the cells the extra power we're demanding from them.

All of this is far more complex than described here, but for the sake of brevity and for the purpose of this book, it's a good foundation.

Where Things Go Wrong

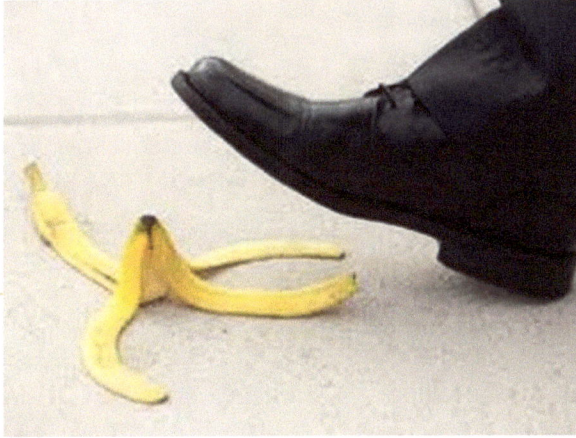

The body is an amazing structure, constantly making the adjustments needed to keep itself in *homeostasis* or perfect balance. Given the opportunity and the right tools, the body will always move in the direction of greater health by protecting the cells, detecting threats, repairing damage and replacing cells that are beyond repair.

The factors that cause this perfect system to break down can be divided into two broad categories: External Influences and Programming.

External Influences

We'll talk about external influences first, because there are a plethora of things outside of us that cause enormous damage inside.

The first thing is *oxidation*. What is oxidation? That's right, it's rust. Just like patio furniture left outside, our cells can rust.

Cellular rust is arguably the most common cause of dysfunction in the body leading to a host of diseases and conditions that shorten life and drain the quality right out of it. Scientists and the medical community refer to cellular rust as *oxidative stress*, and it does the same thing to your cells that it does to your pool lounger, it eats away at the integrity of the structure until the entire thing is weakened and ultimately unable to function. It becomes garbage, and like the chair, it has to be eliminated. Collecting and getting rid of all this garbage puts a burden on the excretory, respiratory, lymphatic and urinary systems of the body which collectively form the body's "waste management" system.

Free Radicals

Free radicals are a huge contributor to the rust. There has been a lot of talk about free radicals in the past twenty years or so and most people understand they damage healthy cells.

At the most basic level, free radicals are simply atoms on a mission. The atom has lost an electron and is therefore out of balance. Because all things in nature move toward balance, the damaged atom "steals" an electron from a neighbor and goes on its way. Now the atom from which the electron was stolen is out of balance, so *it* steals an electron from a neighbor and the process goes on and on. Each time an electron is stolen it creates oxidative stress or rust.

Multiply this process by the millions of times it repeats itself and you can begin to see how that would cause wide-spread damage throughout the body. The number of free radicals present in the body at any given time is estimated to be *one sextillion* (that's a "1" with *twenty-one* zeros).

The extent of the damage free radicals cause is determined by what kind of molecule they steal electrons from. An electron swiped from a glucose molecule won't cause as much damage as one taken from a DNA molecule.

Free radicals aren't choosy; they'll take any available electron to stabilize themselves. In the case of a DNA molecule, this can cause the DNA to mutate and cause disease in the body. There is strong evidence that cancer is formed this way.

So where do free radicals come from? Great question! Free radicals come from several places, including ourselves.

They are a natural by-product of cellular function, so if you have living cells, you have free radicals. They can also be created through exposure to environmental toxins, including radiation, ingested in foods we eat, through skin contact with chemicals, they can even be inhaled. In an ironic twist, it's been found that free radicals can even be created by the very supplements we take to improve our health.

Viruses

Viruses are particularly sneaky. When a virus invades the body, it secretes enzymes that make a hole in the cell wall. Once the cell is vulnerable, the virus then slips into the cell and accesses the DNA to replicate itself. Disguised as a resident cell, the virus can slip right past the army of *lymphocytes* which constantly scan the body and destroy invaders.

Chemical Toxins

Chemical toxins are all around us. It may come as a surprise to learn that often the place with the most toxins and poorest air quality is our homes. Our homes are a "toxic soup" of the various chemicals we use for cleaning, killing bugs, "freshening" the air, etc.

Every day, we expose ourselves and our families to chemicals that would require the use of protective gear if used in the workplace.

Take a look under your kitchen sink and read the labels of the products you find there, it can be an eye-opening experience. When you're done there, go look in your bathroom cabinet. When we did this we found out we were bathing our baby in *formaldehyde* which was an ingredient in the extremely popular brand of baby wash we used, talk about a shock!

The good news is there are places to get safer, natural cleaners and personal care products. We've used them in our own home for several years now (since the formaldehyde incident) and can easily say they are just as (and in a lot of cases, even more) effective as the toxic ones sold in stores. The places to get them are listed at the back of the book.

Radiation

Radiation is another environmental factor that can do a lot of damage. Radiation occurs naturally and can't be avoided even bananas emit small levels of radiation. There are some offenders that are worse than others. The next image shows some of the sources of radiation we encounter every day.

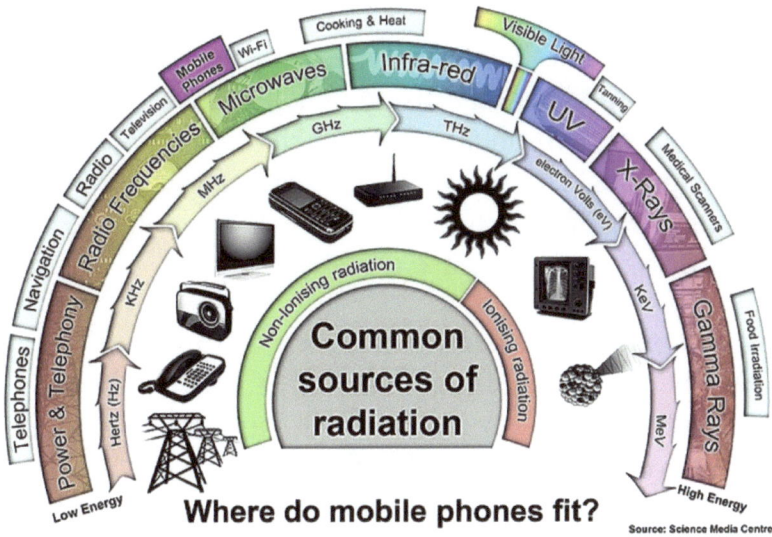

Common sources of radiation

Where do mobile phones fit?

Source: Science Media Centre

Pardon Me....There's a Monster in Your Pocket

Cell phone companies are working very hard to convince us all that the radiation emitted by a cell phone is harmless and very strictly speaking they are correct.

However, an on-going study conducted by Dr. Devra Davis, author of, **Disconnect: The Truth About Cell Phone Radiation**, has shown that while the actual radiation emitted by a cell phone is low, the alternating signal it emits is interfering with DNA repair, reducing sperm counts in men and contributing to cancers.

The greatest harm is caused when we are within six inches of the cell phone's antenna. Considering that a study shows that almost all cell phone users are within are within arm's reach of their phones 23 hours a day (evidently we only tear ourselves away from the phone long enough to shower), we spend several hours per day inside that six inch danger zone. Men often carry their phones in a pocket or belt holder, so they are at greater risk than a woman who carries her phone in her purse. People who hold the phone to their ear are at more risk than people who use a headset.

The picture on the next page shows the exposure that happens when a child holds a cell phone to her ear. The bones in a child's skull are thinner than those of an adult, so they are at even greater risk. After reading Dr. Davis's material, and seeing that picture, we made the decision to continue to use our cell phones, but we treat them more like loaded guns than toys. We keep them at as much distance as possible, use a headset (not a bluetooth) and the little ones are NEVER allowed to touch or play with them.

The Environmental Health Trust is working tirelessly to bring the dangers to light, but of course, the mobile phone industry is enormous and billions of dollars are at stake. The truth will usually find a way to surface and Dr. Davis's findings are slowly getting the attention of the mainstream media. You can hear what she has to say at http://environmentalhealthtrust.org.

"Davis makes a strong case in her book that we've underplayed the possible threat from cell phones for too long... Time and again, she shows the way that industry has been able to twist science just enough to stave off the possibility of any regulation."

- *TIME Magazine*

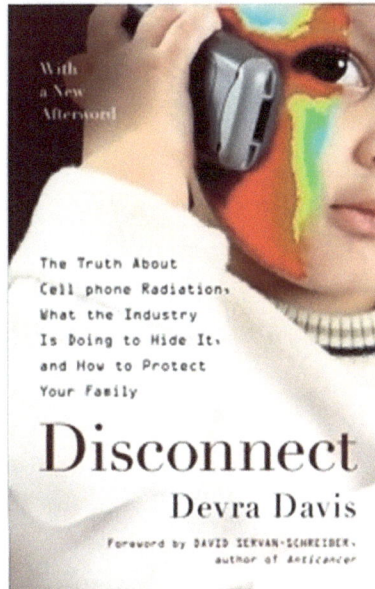

With a New Afterword

The Truth About Cell phone Radiation, What the Industry Is Doing to Hide It, and How to Protect Your Family

Disconnect

Devra Davis

Foreword by DAVID SERVAN-SCHREIBER, author of Anticancer

The Washington Post
The New York Times
C-SPAN
MercuryNews.com
msnbc
MailOnline
THE WALL STREET JOURNAL
TIME
The Miami Herald
NEW YORK POST
THE GLOBE AND MAIL
CBCnews

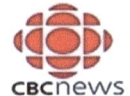

Dead Food

Many people honestly believe they can get all the tools they need for health through a healthy diet.

Unfortunately, that hasn't been true for many years. Because of farming methods that deplete the soil of essential nutrients, it is almost impossible to purchase (or even grow) nutritionally dense foods. In 1977, Dr. Walter Mertz of the US Department of Agriculture made the following statement to Congress:

"In the future, we will not be able to rely anymore on our premise that the consumption of a varied, balanced diet will provide all the essential trace elements, because such a diet will be very difficult to obtain for millions of people."

That future has come to pass. While we can (and should) be careful to consume food that is as fresh and organic as possible, the 2004 edition of McCance and Widdowson's **The Composition of Food** shows an alarming decrease in the essential trace minerals of meat and dairy products compared between levels in 1940 and 2002. Somewhere, Dr. Mertz is saying "I told you so".   Some of the findings include:

Mineral Content of Food
1940 vs 2002

Dairy

Milk	62% less iron
Cheese	70% less calcium
Cheese	70% less magnesium
All	90% less copper

Meat

Magnesium	10% less
Potassium	16% less
Copper	24% less
Phosphorus	28% less
Sodium	30% less
Calcium	41% less
Iron	54% less

Results like these show the difficulty of maintaining health by diet alone. The minerals and trace elements we need are no longer in the soil, so they are not in the plants grown in the soil, therefore they are not in the people and animals that eat the plants that grow in the soil that the minerals and trace elements are not in... whew!!

In a nutshell, just as we are only as healthy as our sickest cell, our food (or the food our food eats) is only as nutritious as the soil in which it grows. It may look great, it can even taste great, but nutritionally it's dead.

Glycation

Gly...what? *Glycation* may be a new term, but the problem has been around for a long time and is getting worse every day. Glycation occurs when *glucose* or sugar found in foods attaches itself to the proteins in our DNA and causes it to malfunction. Picture the way little quagga mussels attach themselves to boats or anything exposed to lake water, glucose does something very similar and just as difficult to repair.

As we age, glycation becomes much harder to repair. This makes prevention extremely important, so pay close attention to the sugar content of all the foods you eat, particularly processed foods. Very often foods labeled "fat free" will contain enormous amounts of sugar to improve the taste.

The Enemy Within...Programming

What we've talked about so far have been just a thumbnail sketch of the external threats our bodies must face and cope with every day. Now we'll talk about the dirty trick nature itself has in store for each of us.

To put this into perspective, let's use a computer analogy.

Most of us have had the experience of purchasing a computer that worked great for a certain amount of time then unexplainably stopped working. A trip to the computer repair shop probably gave you a new phrase for your computer vocabulary; *planned obsolescence.*

Planned obsolescence means your computer was designed to quit working after a set amount of time. It's a sneaky marketing move by computer companies to ensure steady sales, but that is a topic for another time.

Nature has its own form of planned obsolescence. As we age, the body stops or slows down producing things that help us regenerate. We were all born with an expiration date. It sounds harsh, but on a logical level, it's an effective way of controlling the population so there are enough resources for the young.

The very good news on this front is there has been an amazing breakthrough in technology that can give each of us the ability to override this programming.

Since you are now probably wondering what you can do to extend your "shelf life", we'll talk about that next.

Mom Was Right

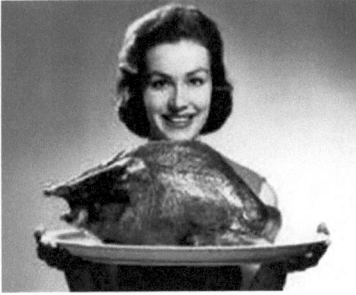

The "common sense" things that most of us already know about are still very important.

We all need to eat a healthy diet, drink water, get plenty of exercise, spend some time in the sunshine and fresh air, and get a good night's sleep.

Here is how science backs up some of Mom's advice:

Healthy Diet

In the "Where Things go Wrong" section, we talked about dead food. Very little of what we can purchase in grocery stores packs the nutrition it did a few generations ago. There are also more unhealthy ingredients being added to preserve the shelf-life of processed foods.

Some communities are known as "food deserts" meaning the residents don't have access to fresh produce, instead, they have to do most of their food shopping from convenience stores and gas stations.

It's important to find trustworthy sources of food. Many organic gardeners are careful to maintain the health of the soil in order to produce healthy plants that don't need artificial supplements and pesticides.

There is a grassroots effort in the U.S. that is gaining momentum called *Community Supported Agriculture* (CSA). Community Supported Agriculture is growing in popularity as more people take an active interest in the source of their daily food. The premise is that people "pre-order" locally grown food. This allows farmers to produce what people want in "just enough" quantities. Throughout the season, the farmer fills the orders.

By taking the guesswork out of what should be planted and in what quantities, farmers are able to work more efficiently and save the money that would be lost in surplus produce that goes to waste. Families benefit because it provides a consistent source of fresh produce which has been grown locally. Information about how to find a CSA in your area is located in the back of this book

Perhaps the most trustworthy source of healthy produce is your own backyard (or patio). Gardening provides the extra benefits of sunshine, fresh air and exercise as well as healthy food. If space is an issue, there is a terrific primer available through Amazon that will show you how to make the most of whatever space you have. It's called *Tips on Potting Veggies in Small Spaces* and is a quick read packed with great information for the small or new gardener. The URL to get it is at the back of the book.

Water

Water could be called the body's Swiss Army Knife, it serves as an essential tool for many critical functions in the body. Water carries oxygen and nutrients to the cells and carries away waste products. It cushions the joints, regulates body temperature, protects vital organs and dissolves minerals and nutrients to make them available to the body.

A healthy body will keep itself hydrated by stimulating thirst. A 1% drop in the body's water reserves will cause thirst.

There is a small division in the medical community over the amount and source of water we need every day. The standard 64 ounces a day has been challenged with a new recommendation being about 50 ounces for a healthy adult. The recommended source used to be that it should be pure water, the new thinking says it can be a combination of water and other water based drinks such as tea and coffee. All sides are in agreement, however, that we all need water every day.

Exercise

After a decade of research into the subject, the US Dept. of Health and Human Services published a guide in 2008 stating that most adults need an average of 2 1/2 hours of moderate exercise per week.

The Department recommends a combination of endurance (aerobic) and resistance (muscle training) activities and notes that the benefits of exercise are cumulative so any activity is better than none at all.

The guide also states that the benefits of exercise far outweigh the risk of injury. The URL to the guide in its entirety is at the back of the book.

Sunshine

There has been a huge push to warn people of the dangers of sun exposure. Even school children are being taught to "Slap, Slip, Slop" (Slap on a hat, Slip on a long-sleeved shirt and Slop on some sunscreen). This advice needs to be taken in moderation. Excessive sun exposure *is* very damaging and has been clearly linked to skin cancer.

However, our fanatical avoidance of the sun has resulted in wide-spread Vitamin D deficiency and depression. A whopping 90% of people tested in the US were vitamin D deficient.

Vitamin D has several forms. The form found in milk and other dairy products is the D2 variety. We've all seen the commercials for the benefits consuming dairy products. What the dairy industry doesn't tell us is that D2 is poorly absorbed by the body and can actually be toxic. The form we need is *vitamin D3*. Researchers have established that *every* cell in the body absolutely requires vitamin D3 to function properly.

Vitamin D3 is found in some foods, particularly salmon and other "fatty" fish. The very best source however is direct sunlight. That means outdoors, not inside with the blinds open because window glass absorbs and deflects too many of the beneficial rays.

Basking in the sun for about 15 minutes three times a week is the current recommendation to provide an adequate supply of D3; after that, "slap, slip, slop" is good advice.

Exposure to sunlight also affects hormone production. When sunlight enters the brain via the optic nerve, it stimulates the pituitary, pineal and hypothalamus glands in the brain. These glands are responsible for a host of body functions including regulating temperature, thirst, hunger, blood pressure, immune response, and secreting the hormones that control proper sexual development and mood.

This explains why Seasonal Affective Disorder (SAD) shows up during the time of year when the days are shortest and why blood pressure increases as a person moves farther away from the equator and the hours of daylight are decreased.

Fresh Air

As we learned in the last section, indoor air is often the most polluted. We build "tiny boxes" to live in then fill the air inside these boxes with harmful chemicals by spraying things like cleaners, air fresheners, perfumes, deodorants, etc.

Even things we don't spray release toxins into the air. Dishwasher detergent, for example, contains bleach and lye which are released into the air as the dishwasher runs. If you'll notice the next time you run a load of dishes, you can smell the bleach. It's a sad truth that many of us associate the smell of bleach with "clean"; it should be associated with "dangerous chemical".

Outdoor air comes in two varieties: positively charged and negatively charged (we're talking about the ions in the air here). Usually "positive" is a good thing, but not in this case. When it comes to air, we need exposure to the negatively charged variety.

Negatively charged ions promote feelings of relaxation and well-being. They lower the body's resting heart rate and help the *cilia* - the little hair-like structures in the respiratory system that "sweep" it clean- function more efficiently.

Good places to find negatively charged ions are at the beach and after a thunderstorm. Whenever you have an opportunity, spend as much time as you can in negatively charged air.

Sleep

It wouldn't be much of a stretch to say that, as a whole, we are a sleep-deprived people.

We live in a fast-paced world and the struggle to keep up is one we all fight to some degree. We reward the "go-getters" who go to great lengths to constantly raise the bar for being productive and label the rest as "lazy". What we're just finding out, though, is those "go-getters" are paying a terrible price when they sacrifice sleep.

During sleep, the body takes advantage of the break to carry out major restorative functions: tissues are repaired, muscles grow, protein is synthesized and growth hormone is released. In a Harvard study which demonstrated the importance of sleep, it was found the immune systems of the study animals that had been deprived of sleep shut down completely and the animals died within a short period of time.

It's been common wisdom that we need 6-8 hours of restful sleep each night.

A more recent discovery reveals that *when* we sleep is important also. The body has an internal clock which establishes our *circadian rhythm*. We won't go into much detail here, but the clock is located in the hypothalamus (the same one we talked about in the "sunshine" section). The clock is regulated or "set" by exposure to light and darkness.

During times of darkness, the body rests and restores itself. During periods of light, it produces energy for activity. It's been discovered that the body does the bulk of its restorative work between the hours of 10:00pm and 2:00am.

You can see what a problem this creates over time for people whose jobs require them to work during these hours. They are accumulating a deficit that just gets larger and larger and moves the potential for huge health consequences into the future...the future they probably plan to spend doing the things they enjoy.

The Game Changer

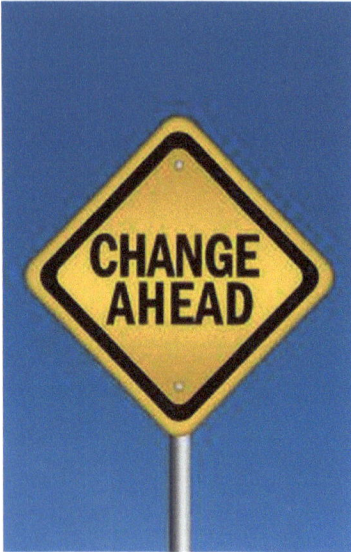

We saved the best for last because there has very recently been a breakthrough in technology that is stirring a great deal of excitement in the world of science. It will soon be widely known and you'll have the advantage of having heard it first!

That sounds like hype, but when you get through reading this section, we think you will agree.

Is Aging Becoming a Choice?

Chronological aging is certain. Time moves forward and we become one day older every day that we live.

However, *cellular aging* and the decline and disease that come with it, is becoming optional.

Just a few short years ago, the ability to stop or reverse cellular aging was pure theory. Advancements moved it into the realm of possibility and a very recent breakthrough has turned it from a possibility into a probability and put it into the hands of people everywhere.

You and I and everyone we know can -at the very least- slow down the process that is bringing each of us closer to our "expiration date" every day.

Because the technology that makes this possible is very new, we don't have case studies that demonstrate the new life-expectancy of people who choose to slow down the aging process. We do know, however that scientists have been able to create what they refer to as "immortal cells". These are human cells that, under optimum conditions in a laboratory, have been regenerating themselves for many years and show no signs of decline or aging.

There is a lot of enthusiasm in the scientific community about how this will change the way we age.

Miraculous Messengers

Remember the redox signaling molecules that were thought to simply be a by-product of ATP production? Someday, future generations are going to laugh at that idea like we laugh at the "DDT is good for me" idea today.

We won't go into the back story of how scientists came to study these "waste products" which opened up an entirely new field of study called *Redox Biochemistry*. The important thing is what they discovered. Remember the objectives of a cell:

1. Protect itself from harm

2. Detect damage

3. Repair the damage if possible

4. Replace cells that are beyond repair

Redox signaling molecules are *critical* to the protection of cells, the detection of damage and the repair or replacement of damaged cells. At birth these cells are functioning at 100%, that's why babies and young children have so much energy and can heal so quickly. At about age 12, efficiency starts to decrease until by the time we are 70 or so, they are only working at about 10%. This is the reason we tire faster and it takes longer to heal from illness or injuries as we age.

Remember that redox signaling molecules are produced in pairs. In order to function properly both are needed. The first molecule, the *reduced species* or *(RS)* is tasked with **Antioxidant Activation.**

It would be hard to find someone who *hasn't* heard of antioxidants. Their ability to neutralize free radicals is almost the stuff of legends and supplement companies are tripping over themselves to spread the word about the ORAC *(oxygen radical absorbance capacity)* value of their product.

They have it half right.

Antioxidants *are* important in the battle against free radicals.

The other half of the story is that without a sufficient amount of redox signaling molecules to *activate* the antioxidants, a person may as well be eating M & M's. By the time most of us are concerned enough about our health to be taking antioxidant supplements, we only have enough redox signaling molecule efficiency to activate a small fraction of them. Antioxidants without RS to activate them are about as useful as a light bulb with no source of electricity.

Antioxidants are not created equal

Most of the antioxidants available for purchase are derived from plants. Technically, they may have great free radical-fighting properties (that's the ORAC score that's talked about all the time), but the molecules are very large; 200 atoms wide and often larger. This makes it impossible for them to go through the cell wall. They can only have an effect on free radicals *outside* the cells.

Nature is wise and has given the body the ability to produce its own (native) antioxidants called *superoxides.* Superoxides are far more powerful than any over the counter antioxidant supplement or juice. *Glutathione, super oxide dismutase (SOD)* and *catalase* are extremely powerful antioxidants made even more effective by redox signaling molecules.

Each antioxidant in over the counter supplements can only neutralize one free radical by giving up an electron, then *it* becomes a free radical.

Individual superoxides produced by the body neutralize approximately 70 million free radicals every day. They are long-lived and when they are spent, they create more superoxides as a last contribution before they die.

Just as a note, you will see supplements containing the native antioxidants, particularly glutathion, on the market. The problem to date has been finding a way to bind the antioxidants so they aren't destroyed when they come into contact with stomach acid. You'll want to check the *bioavailability* (how much of it is actually able to be absorbed and used by the body) of any supplements you are considering purchasing.

When activated by RS, the superoxides, are 500-800% more effective; giving them the ability to neutralize hundreds of millions of free radicals. If you remember that the body is dealing with one-sextillion free radicals every day, you can see that superoxides activated by RS are the only way to even make a dent in the number of free radicals.

Communicators

The second molecule in the set, *reactive oxygen species* or (ROS) is tasked with **cellular communication**. Our bodies are extremely complex information systems. Millions of messages are being sent and received continually to keep everything functioning.

As a quick demonstration, scratch your nose with your index finger. Now consider how many messages had to go from your brain to your arm to raise it to your nose. More messages had to go to your finger to tell it to extend and find your nose. Even more messages had to be sent and received to control the amount of pressure used and still more to control the up and down movement as you scratched. A whole new set of messages were generated to tell your finger to stop and for your arm to return to its original position.

This is just a small example. Imagine the complexity of the messages that allow us to write a grocery list, engage in a sport, or pick up a penny on the ground.

For those who like a challenge, read the following:

7H15 M3554G3 53RV35 70 PROV3 HOW 0UR M1ND5 C4N DO 4M4Z1NG 7H1NG5. 1MPR3551V3 7H1NG5! 1N 7H3 B3G1NN1NG 17 WA5 H4RD BU7 N0W, 0N 7H15 L1N3 Y0UR M1ND I5 R34D1NG 17 4U70M471C4LLY.

If scientists had been scanning your brain while it figured out the "code" in the message above and adapted to it, they would have seen your brain literally light up as it sent messages back and forth at lightning speed. This entire process relies on cellular communication and cellular communication relies on ROS.

 The other function of ROS is immune response. The ROS are "first responders" that attack bacteria, viruses or other invaders on contact. They then signal the immune system and tell it to mobilize the army of lymphocytes to crush the invasion.

The molecules must co-exist in perfect balance because ROS kills invaders with oxygen then RS sweeps in and neutralizes the oxidation this produces.

What we know today about redox signaling molecules and what they do is just the tip of the iceberg. There are strong initial findings that redox signaling molecules play a very important role in genetic expression and protecting the telomere ends that keep our DNA strands in perfect form. Every time the cell divides, the telomere becomes a little shorter. When it reaches a certain length, the cell will no longer be able to divide. There is a strong link between short telomeres and cancer (and the odds of dying of cancer) so there is a great deal of interest in this aspect of the research.

Here's the Important Part

Until just a few years ago, the downside of Redox Biochemistry has been that while we gained an understanding of how crucial the molecules are, there was nothing we could do to give the body more of them. For over seventeen years scientists tried to re-create the molecules outside of the body using various means. It became the "it can't be done" challenge of the time.

There was an early breakthrough several years ago when the first molecules were created in a lab by breaking apart and recombining the atoms found in salt water. Unfortunately, the molecules were extremely unstable and reverted back to their original form in just a few minutes.

The researchers then developed a small machine that could create the molecules for immediate use and began testing the effect of the created molecules with some volunteers.

The volunteers in the study saw an almost immediate benefit (within two weeks) after starting a regimen of drinking two ounces of the molecule solution twice a day. Everyone in the test group told of changes they had noticed. Scars were disappearing, people had more energy, colds sputtered and died within a few hours of onset. The reports went on and on.

One completely unexpected benefit was reported by those in the test group who happened to be athletes. They reported their endurance had increased dramatically. Performance studies in the lab later showed this to be true; the athletes in the study increased their *ventilatory threshold* (the time it takes to hit the "runner's wall") by 12%. Just to demonstrate how significant this is, illegal performance enhancing drugs only increase the ventilatory threshold by about 2%.

In a competition where the difference between winning or being an "also ran" is often just a fraction of a second, a 12% increase is monumental.

The test group using the redox signaling molecules had a huge *fatty acid mobilization* even before they began to exercise. This gave their bodies the perfect fuel for the strenuous workouts that were part of the study. The researchers found the athletes also had far less post-workout soreness and recovered very quickly.

The team knew they were on to a discovery that needed to be available more easily to more people so the search continued for a way to stabilize the molecules.

Finally, Dr. Gary Samuelson, an Atomic Physicist, made the final breakthrough. He and his team developed a process that stabilized the solution and kept it in perfect form for two years.

The team he was working with submitted an *Indication of New Drug* report to the FDA then sent the solution for toxicity testing as a first step for FDA approval.

After spending over five million dollars in testing, the results came back that the solution caused absolutely zero inflammatory response in any of the tests. A funny thing happened while they were trying to establish the lethal dose as required by the FDA; they kept giving the animals they were using more and more of the solution, watching for signs of toxicity, but the animals just kept getting healthier and healthier.

The team was ecstatic! The doors this could open for new treatments and health benefits were endless! All they needed now was a way to distribute it.

The story takes a twist here. The team presented the perfected solution to a large pharmaceutical company and offered to sell it to them. The company had its in-house researchers go through every bit of documentation on it, and then offered a huge amount of money to buy the rights to the research.

The team was delirious with happiness for a moment; they would finally make back all the money they had spent developing it and then some.

However, the pharmaceutical company had one caveat: they were to immediately withdraw all the solution that had been given to the volunteers and turn over all copies of the research results.

At that point, the team realized the company was not offering to buy the solution to distribute it; they wanted to buy it to suppress it.

Because they had seen the effects the molecules had produced, and watched their volunteers' lives change, they decided they couldn't allow that to happen (this is the good part). They swallowed hard and went back to the pharmaceutical company and told them "no deal".

They said "no" to the payout and "yes" to the people!

Then they rolled up their collective sleeves and went to work figuring out how to get the solution into the hands of the people who needed it by themselves.

Headed up by Verdis Norton and James Pack, who had both had extremely successful corporate careers, they formed a company and now, the molecules, in their perfect *bioavailable* form, are available to everyone.

The huge take-away from Redox Biochemistry research is that for the first time in the history of mankind, we have a health technology that allows us to restore the very building blocks of youth, health and endurance.

Age is becoming just a number; and that number means less every day.

See the resource pages to find out how to put these amazing molecules to work for you.

Putting it All Together

Knowledge is power...

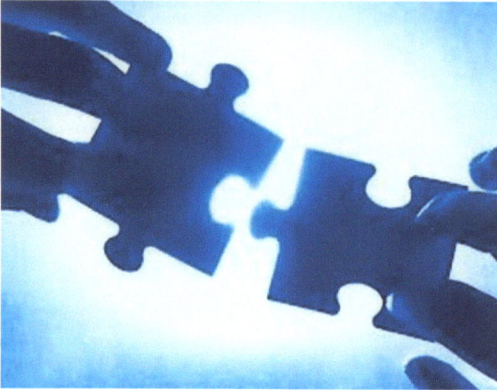

Are You in the 10% Group?

We think you will agree that knowledge
is *potential* power....**applied** knowledge is power.

Now that you know about the building blocks of health and
how they work, the question is what will you do with the
knowledge? Statistics say that 90% of the people who read
this will do nothing. But if you're one of the 10%, you want
this information to change your life and you'll take the action
to make it happen. Here's how you can apply what you
know to what you do every day and get the maximum
advantage.

Start Slowly...Eating an Elephant

The old joke, *how do you eat an elephant?...one bite at a time!* has a lot of wisdom in it.

Change is hard but studies have shown that people who make small changes over a period of time are more likely to continue and experience a greater benefit than people who try to make sweeping changes all at once. It's best to create a personal program for yourself, one that you can maintain until it becomes a habit.

Manage Your Expectations

A lot of people have a specific health goal in mind, they are trying to solve a particular problem or get a specific benefit.

While goals are generally good, it's important to know that *your* priorities are not necessarily *your body's* priorities. In truth, your body has its own "to do" list and it will use the materials you provide to accomplish what *it* has set as a priority.

Knowing this, it's important to pay attention to notice little improvements in areas you may not expect to see them. The "easy" fixes will be made first, so you may notice things like sleeping better at night and waking more refreshed. It may be an increase of energy during the day or improved memory. Whatever the little fixes are, make sure to make note of them so you can get an idea of the progress you're making.

Taking Out the Trash

Your body does an amazing job of doing what it can with what it has.

That means that as you start providing it with high quality materials, it's going to start building and repairing in earnest.

Just like the rusty pool chair that had to go to the dump, your cells that need to be replaced will start dying off so new ones can take their place. All this "cellular garbage" has to go somewhere and that "somewhere" is places like your liver and kidneys so it can be eliminated.

Because there is so much garbage that needs to be handled, you will probably experience a "detox" period soon after you start. Everyone responds differently, so it's hard to say what you may experience during the detox, but it generally includes feeling fatigued. The short explanation for this is your body wants you to sleep so it can focus on "cleaning house" instead of providing energy for physical activity.

One of the most dramatic stories I've ever heard about someone detoxing is about a person who had smoked menthol cigarettes for many years. As her body began to detox, she had little bumps pop out all over her skin. Inside each of the bumps was a small fragment of the fiberglass that menthol cigarettes contain. That is an amazing example of how far the body will go to heal itself when it's given the ability to do so.

Starting slowly will help your body detox more gradually. You can give it a hand by supporting it with great nutrition. Some people also benefit from using one of the various cleansing products available. Most of these will be in the form of supplements and teas or drinks made with a mixture of soothing and detoxifying herbs.

Stick With It

The most important part of your personal program is your commitment to it. It's vital to stick with it until it becomes habit, then to maintain that habit for life.

Oddly enough, the point where some people have quit isn't when the going got hard, like during the detox period; they quit *when they felt better*!!! Somehow the thought formed that because they felt better and had received all the great benefits they needed, they didn't need to continue their health program. It sounds ridiculous, but it can happen. That's why the commitment part is so important.

Don't quit if you feel bad for a short time and *definitely* don't quit when you start feeling great!

The Next Step

What will applying the things you've learned in this book do for you? The only way to find out is to try them. Make a few lifestyle changes, provide your body with nutritious food, walk more, enjoy some sunshine and fresh air!

Be sure to include redox signaling molecules in your action plan. They will "power up" everything else you're doing to give you the greatest benefit from all of it.

If you want to learn more about them, head to the companion website for this book at www.youthhealthendurance.com. We've gathered some of the best research there for you.

The Brains Behind the Book

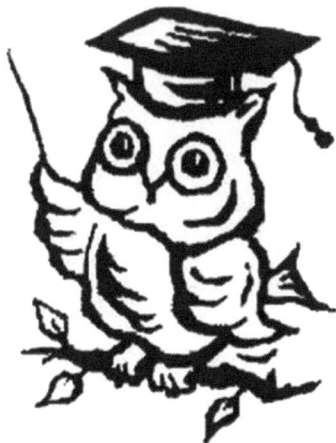

All the information in this book comes from real-life heroes; the people who have invested the time, money, and other resources to make these discoveries. Our goal in writing this book for you was to give a brief overview of some of the important things that have come to light in recent years.

It is our hope that we have planted a seed of curiosity, an urge to learn more. For that reason, all the sources that contributed information for the writing of this book are listed in this section.

When you read them for yourself, you'll have a deeper understanding of how much control we really have to influence the state of our health.

The sources for some of the products and books we talked about are listed first. These are the places we found them, you may find others. If you find a great source for something, hop over to the website for this book at http://www.youthhealthendurance.com and let everyone know.

The sources of information are listed also. Again, this is in no way an exhaustive list. If you see an article somewhere that helps you, chances are it will help someone else too; head to the website and tell us about it...don't forget to post a link so we can all read it!

To your health,

The Authors

Where to Get Things

As we find other sources of supply we will update the

website for this book

at http://youthhealthendurance.com Be sure to check

it out!

Redox Signaling Molecules

You can learn more and order redox signaling molecules from:

This will most likely be the only place to ever get these because the process for creating and stabilizing them is heavily patented (thirty-one patents and counting). When you get to the site, take a few minutes and watch some of the videos and read some of the research for yourself. You'll find all the independent scientific verifications and study results here too.

Non-toxic Household Cleaners

When we first decided to "detox" our house, we tried making our own cleaners. There are plenty of people who swear by this and you may want to try it for yourself. You can find some ideas at www.earthjustice.org A quick online search will give you dozens of sites for more recipes.

We wanted something with a little more "muscle" so we turned to the "green cleaners" at the store. Some people love them, and they were satisfactory for light cleaning. We have industrial-strength kids and dogs that make epic messes and stains so we had to keep searching for something more effective.

There are some non-toxic household cleaners available here: www.eartheasy.com/green-home We have not used them, but others have told us they use them all the time and like them a lot. If you order from here, give us a review on the website at www.youthhealthendurance.com so other people can benefit from your experience.

We love the products at www.melaleuca.com It's a members-only store, a membership costs $29 for a year. If you click the small link at the top of their webpage that says "contact us", the company will give you the name of someone who can help you set up your shopping account. They offer direct memberships or for deeper discounts, you can choose to be become a preferred member. The person who helps you will explain the difference. Setting up an account is a little bit of a nuisance, but it was worth it to us because the products are very effective. These are the ones we've used exclusively for over two years.

We've also used products from www.amway.com and like them much better than the ones available at the store. If you don't want to have someone contact you and go through the process of setting up an account, you can shop directly from this site. Their prices are reasonable, but the shipping costs are rather high. You may have a different experience depending on where you live.

Whether you mix them up yourself or order from a company or a combination of both, the important thing is to find something that works best for you and start eliminating the "toxic soup" in your home.

Negative Ion Generators

You can find negative ion generators for you home and more information on what negative ions do at www.surroundair.com/negative-ions.htm

Just as a thought; while negative ions are very beneficial, negative ion generators can create a strong electromagnetic field (EMF) in their immediate area. You may want to educate yourself on EMF's before you decide to bring one into your home.

Healthy Diet

Community supported agriculture programs in your area can be found at: www.localharvest.org/csa/

Tips on Potting Veggies in Small Spaces is available at www.amazon.com if you search it by the title, you'll find it.

The Composition of Food is also available at www.amazon.com

http://www.dinnergarden.org is a wonderful place with an important mission. They have been quietly fighting hunger by teaching people how to grow food in their own space using containers that most of us just throw away. They also provide seeds at no cost to families in need. They support themselves through the sale of their awesome cookbook. We donate a percentage of the proceeds from the sale of this book to them and hope you will find it in your heart to help them out too.

Sources of Information

Cell Phone Dangers

The Environmental Health Trust- Dr. Derva Davis
www.environmentalhealthtrust.org

Water

Water as an Essential Nutrient: The Physiological Basis of Hydration- European Journal of Clinical Nutrition volume 64
www.nature.com

Exercise

2008 Physical Activity Guidelines for Americans -US
Department of Health and Human Services
www.health.gov/paguidelines

Sleep

Harvard study www.healthysleep.med.harvard.edu

Sunshine

Photobiology: The Biological Impact of Sunlight on Health
and Infection Control www.phoenixprojectfoundation.us

Fresh Air

The Influence of Negative Air Ions on Human Performance
and Mood http://hfs.sagepub.com/content/23/5/633.short

Redox Signaling Molecules
(apologies for the small font, most of these reports have very long names)

Critical Care 10(208) (2006), "Reactive oxygen species: toxic molecules or spark of life?", Shelden Magder (http://ccforum.com/content/10/1/208).

Biochemical Pharmacology 70 (2005) 811-823, "Redox regulation: A new challenge for pharmacology", Daniel Frein, Stefan Schildknecht (http://www.ncbi.nlm.nih.gov/pubmed/15899473).

J Radiat Res (Tokyo 2004) 45(3) 357-72 "Oxidative stress, radiation-adaptive responses, and aging", Miura Y. (http://www.ncbi.nlm.nih.gov/pubmed/15613781).

J Cell Bio: minireview, "Specificity in reactive oxidant signaling: think globally, act locally", Lance S. Terada (http://www.ncbi.nlm.nih.gov/pubmed/16923830).

www.ingramcontent.com/pod-product-compliance
Lightning Source LLC
Chambersburg PA
CBHW041222270326
41933CB00001B/5

* 9 7 8 0 6 1 5 7 0 1 6 3 9 *